Blood Type O Diet Cookbook

I0427206

Becky Shelby

Table of Contents

Introduction

Within the rhythm of our everyday lives, there lies a profound connection, often overlooked in the hustle and bustle. This cookbook, crafted with utmost care and genuine intent, extends an invitation to rediscover that connection – a connection between our bodies and the nourishment that sustains us. It is an ode to those with blood type O, an acknowledgment that what we consume is more than mere sustenance; it's a language our bodies speak.

In the delicate tapestry of these pages, envision not just a collection of recipes, but rather a journey toward wellness, a journey designed to align with the principles of the Blood Type O Diet. This culinary adventure seeks to be a guide, a companion as you navigate the intricate dance between the ingredients on your plate and the very essence of your being.

Here, you won't find a mere compilation of dishes; instead, each recipe is a reflection of passion, understanding, and a deep respect for the connection between nutrition and vitality. As you explore these culinary creations, consider it an exploration of self-love and a commitment to nurturing the extraordinary vessel that is your body.

So, within these chapters, let the kitchen become a sanctuary, and let each meal be an affirmation of your commitment to well-being. This cookbook is an offering, a reminder that each bite can be an act of self-love and a celebration of the uniqueness inherent in every blood type O individual.

Here's to the intentional creation of nourishing meals, to savoring the richness of life, and to fostering a profound connection with your own well-being. May this cookbook be a guide on your journey to vibrant health, reminding you that, with each mindful and delicious bite, you're choosing to embrace a healthier, more vibrant version of yourself. Enjoy this culinary exploration; you've earned it.

Understanding The Blood Type O Diet

The Blood Type O Diet, popularized by Dr. Peter J. D'Adamo, is a nutritional approach that tailors dietary recommendations based on an individual's blood type. According to this theory, blood type O individuals are believed to thrive on a diet reminiscent of their ancestors, who were presumed to be hunter-gatherers.

The Basics

1. Protein Emphasis:

   - Meat and Poultry: Advocates of the Blood Type O Diet suggest that individuals with blood type O tend to do well with animal proteins, particularly lean meats such as beef, lamb, and poultry.

   - Fish: Fish, particularly those rich in omega-3 fatty acids like salmon and mackerel, are often encouraged.

2. Limited Grains:

   - Wheat-Free Grains: The diet recommends minimizing or eliminating wheat and gluten-containing grains. Instead, individuals with blood type O may opt for rice, quinoa, and other gluten-free grains.

3. Fruits and Vegetables:

 - Rich in Vegetables: A diet abundant in vegetables is promoted, with an emphasis on leafy greens, broccoli, and other nutrient-dense options.

 - Moderate Fruits: While fruits are generally encouraged, those with blood type O are often advised to favor fruits like berries, plums, and figs.

4. Dairy Considerations:

 - Limited Dairy: The consumption of dairy, especially milk and cheese, may be limited, as individuals with blood type O are believed to be less tolerant to lactose.

5. Beans and Legumes:

 - Selective Legumes: While some legumes may be included in the diet, others, like lentils and kidney beans, are often suggested to be consumed in moderation.

6. Nuts and Seeds:

 - Healthy Fats: Nuts and seeds, such as walnuts and flaxseeds, are considered beneficial for blood type O individuals.

According to the Blood Type Diet, individuals with blood type O are generally advised to avoid or minimize the consumption of certain foods that are believed to be less compatible with their blood type. It's essential to note that the scientific basis for these recommendations is limited, and individual responses to foods can vary. Before making significant dietary changes, individuals should consult with healthcare professionals. Here are foods often suggested to be avoided for those with blood type O:

Foods to Avoid or Limit for Blood Type O

1. Wheat and Gluten:

   - Wheat-based products, including bread and pasta, are often discouraged. Gluten-containing grains may be less compatible with blood type O.

2. Dairy Products:

   - Some individuals with blood type O are advised to limit dairy consumption, especially milk and certain types of cheese. Lactose intolerance is more common in individuals with blood type O.

3. Certain Grains:

   - Corn and lentils are often mentioned as grains to be consumed in moderation or avoided.

4. Legumes:

   - Certain legumes, such as kidney beans and navy beans, may be recommended in limited quantities.

5. Cabbage and Brussels Sprouts:

   - These vegetables are suggested to be limited, as they may interfere with thyroid function, which could be of particular concern for blood type O individuals.

6. Cauliflower and Mustard Greens:

   - These cruciferous vegetables are sometimes advised to be consumed in moderation.

7. Certain Fruits:

   - Blood type O individuals may be encouraged to limit their intake of oranges and melons.

8. Processed and High-Sugar Foods:

   - Processed and sugary foods are generally discouraged, as they may contribute to weight gain and other health issues.

9. Caffeine and Alcohol:

   - Coffee and black tea, as well as alcoholic beverages, are often recommended in moderation.

It's important to emphasize that individual responses to foods can vary, and not all individuals with blood type O will experience the same reactions to these foods. Some people may thrive on a diet that aligns with the Blood Type O recommendations, while others may not see significant benefits. However, before making substantial changes to one's diet based on blood type or any other dietary theory, it is advisable to consult with healthcare professionals or registered dietitians. These professionals can provide personalized guidance based on an individual's overall health, medical history, and specific nutritional needs.

Key Principles

1. Individual Variations: It's important to note that individual responses to the Blood Type O Diet can vary. Some individuals may experience positive outcomes, while others may not see significant benefits.

2. Exercise Recommendations: Regular physical activity is often encouraged for individuals with blood type O, including activities that combine both aerobic exercise and strength training.

3. Hydration: Staying adequately hydrated is a fundamental aspect of the Blood Type O Diet, with an emphasis on consuming water and herbal teas.

4. Mindful Eating: The diet promotes mindful eating, encouraging individuals to pay attention to how different foods make them feel and adjusting their diet accordingly.

Caution

While the Blood Type O Diet has gained popularity, it's essential to approach it with a critical mindset. Scientific evidence supporting the personalized dietary recommendations based on blood type is limited, and individuals should consult with healthcare professionals or registered dietitians before making significant changes to their diet.

In conclusion, the Blood Type O Diet is a unique nutritional approach that suggests tailoring dietary choices based on blood type. However, individuals should consider their own health status, preferences, and the available scientific evidence before adopting any specific diet plan.

Chapter 1: Breakfast Delights

1. Omelette Extravaganza

A protein-packed breakfast featuring a fluffy omelette filled with spinach and feta, providing essential nutrients to kickstart your day.

Ingredients:

- 3 large eggs

- 1 cup fresh spinach, chopped

- 1/4 cup feta cheese, crumbled

- Salt and pepper to taste

- 1 tablespoon olive oil

Instructions:

1. In a bowl, whisk the eggs until well beaten. Season with salt and pepper.

2. Heat olive oil in a non-stick skillet over medium heat.

3. Add chopped spinach to the skillet and sauté until wilted.

4. Pour the beaten eggs over the spinach and let them set for a moment.

5. Sprinkle crumbled feta cheese evenly over the eggs.

6. Gently lift the edges of the omelette with a spatula, allowing any uncooked eggs to flow underneath.

7. Once the eggs are fully set, fold the omelette in half.

8. Slide the omelette onto a plate, cut in half, and serve hot.

2. Turkey and Vegetable Scramble

A savory and satisfying scramble combining lean ground turkey with a colorful array of vegetables like bell peppers and onions, offering a hearty and nutritious breakfast.

Ingredients:

- 1/2 lb lean ground turkey

- 1 bell pepper, diced

- 1 onion, diced

- 2 cloves garlic, minced

- Salt and pepper to taste

- Fresh herbs for garnish (e.g., parsley or chives)

Instructions:

1. In a skillet over medium heat, cook the ground turkey until browned.

2. Add diced bell pepper and onion to the skillet and sauté until vegetables are tender.

3. Stir in minced garlic and cook for an additional minute.

4. Season with salt and pepper to taste.

5. Garnish with fresh herbs before serving.

3. Energizing Smoothie Bowl

A vibrant and refreshing smoothie bowl featuring a blend of berries, banana, and spinach, topped with chia seeds and sliced almonds for a nutrient-rich start.

Ingredients:

- 1 cup mixed berries (strawberries, blueberries, raspberries)

- 1 ripe banana

- 1 cup fresh spinach

- 1/2 cup almond milk

- 1 tablespoon chia seeds

- 2 tablespoons sliced almonds

Instructions:

1. In a blender, combine berries, banana, spinach, and almond milk.

2. Blend until smooth and creamy.

3. Pour the smoothie into a bowl.

4. Top with chia seeds and sliced almonds.

5. Enjoy with a spoon!

4. Tropical Green Power Bowl

A tropical-inspired breakfast bowl with a base of coconut milk, topped with fresh mango, kiwi, and a sprinkle of pumpkin seeds for a burst of flavors and essential nutrients.

Ingredients:

- 1/2 cup coconut milk

- 1/2 cup fresh mango, diced

- 1/2 cup fresh kiwi, sliced

- 1/4 cup pineapple chunks

- 2 tablespoons shredded coconut

- 1 tablespoon pumpkin seeds

Instructions:

1. Pour coconut milk into a bowl.

2. Arrange mango, kiwi, and pineapple on top of the coconut milk.

3. Sprinkle shredded coconut and pumpkin seeds over the fruit.

4. Dive into this tropical breakfast delight!

5. Quinoa and Spinach Muffins

Wholesome muffins made with quinoa and spinach, offering a unique twist on traditional breakfast options while providing a good balance of protein and fiber.

Ingredients:

- 1 cup cooked quinoa

- 1 cup fresh spinach, finely chopped

- 3 eggs

- 1/2 cup feta cheese, crumbled

- 1/4 cup grated Parmesan cheese

- 1 teaspoon baking powder

- Salt and pepper to taste

Instructions:

1. Preheat the oven to 350°F (175°C). Grease a muffin tin or line with paper liners.

2. In a large bowl, combine cooked quinoa, chopped spinach, eggs, feta cheese, Parmesan cheese, baking powder, salt, and pepper.

3. Mix until well combined.

4. Spoon the mixture into the muffin cups, filling each almost to the top.

5. Bake for 20-25 minutes or until the muffins are set and golden brown.

6. Allow to cool slightly before serving.

6. Almond Flour Banana Muffins

Moist and delicious muffins made with almond flour and ripe bananas, providing a nutrient-dense alternative for those with blood type O.

Ingredients:

- 2 ripe bananas, mashed

- 3 eggs

- 1/2 cup almond flour

- 1/4 cup coconut flour

- 1/4 cup coconut oil, melted

- 1 teaspoon baking soda

- 1/2 teaspoon vanilla extract

- Pinch of salt

- Chopped nuts (optional, for topping)

Instructions:

1. Preheat the oven to 350°F (175°C). Line a muffin tin with paper liners.

2. In a bowl, whisk together mashed bananas, eggs, melted coconut oil, and vanilla extract.

3. In a separate bowl, combine almond flour, coconut flour, baking soda, and a pinch of salt.

4. Mix the dry ingredients into the wet ingredients until well combined.

5. Spoon the batter into the muffin cups, filling each about two-thirds full.

6. If desired, sprinkle chopped nuts on top.

7. Bake for 20-25 minutes or until a toothpick inserted into the center comes out clean.

7. Berry Blast Breakfast Bowl

A colorful bowl featuring a mix of antioxidant-rich berries, coconut yogurt, and a sprinkle of walnuts, creating a delicious and health-conscious breakfast.

Ingredients:

- 1 cup mixed berries (strawberries, blueberries, raspberries)

- 1/2 cup Greek yogurt

- 2 tablespoons granola

- 1 tablespoon honey

- 1 tablespoon chia seeds

- Fresh mint leaves for garnish

Instructions:

1. In a bowl, layer mixed berries and Greek yogurt.

2. Sprinkle granola on top.

3. Drizzle honey over the granola.

4. Sprinkle chia seeds for added texture.

5. Garnish with fresh mint leaves.

6. Dive into this refreshing and nutritious breakfast bowl.

8. Lemon Garlic Chicken Bowl

A savory bowl with grilled chicken seasoned with lemon and garlic, paired with sautéed vegetables like broccoli and zucchini, offering a satisfying and protein-packed morning meal.

Ingredients:

- 1 boneless, skinless chicken breast

- 1 tablespoon olive oil

- 1 teaspoon lemon zest

- 1 clove garlic, minced

- Salt and pepper to taste

- Mixed vegetables (broccoli, bell peppers, zucchini), steamed

Instructions:

1. Season the chicken breast with salt, pepper, lemon zest, and minced garlic.

2. Heat olive oil in a skillet over medium heat.

3. Cook the chicken until golden brown on both sides and cooked through.

4. Slice the chicken and serve over a bed of steamed mixed vegetables.

9. Teriyaki Salmon Quinoa Bowl

A Japanese-inspired bowl with teriyaki-glazed salmon served over a bed of quinoa, complemented by steamed bok choy and sesame seeds for a nutrient-rich breakfast.

Ingredients:

- 1 salmon fillet

- 2 tablespoons teriyaki sauce

- 1 cup cooked quinoa

- Steamed bok choy

- Sesame seeds for garnish

Instructions:

1. Marinate the salmon fillet in teriyaki sauce for at least 15 minutes.

2. Grill or pan-sear the salmon until cooked to your liking.

3. Place cooked quinoa in a bowl.

4. Top with steamed bok choy and the teriyaki salmon.

5. Garnish with sesame seeds before serving.

10. Spinach and Feta Breakfast Wrap

A quick and portable breakfast option featuring a whole-grain wrap filled with scrambled eggs, spinach, and crumbled feta cheese, providing a well-rounded and flavorful start to the day.

Ingredients:

- 2 large eggs, scrambled

- 1 whole-grain wrap

- Handful of fresh spinach

- 2 tablespoons crumbled feta cheese

- Salt and pepper to taste

Instructions:

1. Scramble the eggs in a pan until cooked through.

2. Lay the whole-grain wrap on a flat surface.

3. Arrange fresh spinach on the wrap.

4. Spoon the scrambled eggs onto the spinach.

5. Sprinkle crumbled feta cheese over the eggs.

6. Season with salt and pepper to taste.

7. Roll the wrap and secure with a toothpick if needed.

8. Enjoy this quick and portable breakfast.

Chapter 2: Lunchtime Favorites

1. Grilled Lemon Herb Chicken Bowl

A delightful bowl featuring grilled chicken marinated in a zesty blend of lemon and herbs. Served over a bed of nutrient-rich leafy greens, this dish is a flavorful and protein-packed lunch option for blood type O individuals.

Ingredients:

- 1 boneless, skinless chicken breast

- 1 tablespoon olive oil

- Zest of 1 lemon

- 1 teaspoon dried oregano

- Salt and pepper to taste

- Mixed greens (e.g., spinach, arugula)

Instructions:

1. Preheat a grill or grill pan over medium-high heat.

2. In a bowl, mix olive oil, lemon zest, dried oregano, salt, and pepper to create the marinade.

3. Coat the chicken breast with the marinade.

4. Grill the chicken for about 6-8 minutes per side or until cooked through.

5. Slice the grilled chicken and serve over a bed of mixed greens.

2. Teriyaki Salmon Quinoa Bowl

Teriyaki-glazed salmon takes center stage in this bowl, accompanied by a generous serving of quinoa and steamed bok choy. The combination of flavors and textures makes for a satisfying and well-balanced lunch.

Ingredients:

- 1 salmon fillet

- 2 tablespoons teriyaki sauce

- 1 cup cooked quinoa

- Steamed bok choy

- Sesame seeds for garnish

Instructions:

1. Marinate the salmon fillet in teriyaki sauce for at least 15 minutes.

2. Grill or pan-sear the salmon until cooked to your liking.

3. Place cooked quinoa in a bowl.

4. Top with steamed bok choy and the teriyaki salmon.

5. Garnish with sesame seeds before serving.

3. Greek Salad with Grilled Chicken

A classic Greek salad gets a protein boost with the addition of grilled chicken. Crisp vegetables, Kalamata olives, and feta cheese come together to create a refreshing and fulfilling lunch option for blood type O.

Ingredients:

- 1 boneless, skinless chicken breast

- 1 tablespoon olive oil

- 1 teaspoon dried oregano

- Salt and pepper to taste

- Mixed salad greens

- Cherry tomatoes, halved

- Cucumber, sliced

- Kalamata olives

- Feta cheese, crumbled

- Greek dressing

Instructions:

1. Season the chicken breast with olive oil, dried oregano, salt, and pepper.

2. Grill the chicken until fully cooked, then slice.

3. In a large bowl, combine salad greens, cherry tomatoes, cucumber, Kalamata olives, and feta cheese.

4. Add the grilled chicken slices on top.

5. Drizzle with Greek dressing and toss before serving.

4. Turkey and Avocado Collard Wraps

Delicious and portable, these collard wraps are filled with lean turkey, avocado slices, and a selection of crisp vegetables. A perfect low-carb option for a quick and nutritious lunch.

Ingredients:

- Collard green leaves (large, destemmed)

- 1/2 lb lean ground turkey

- 1 teaspoon cumin

- 1/2 teaspoon paprika

- Salt and pepper to taste

- Avocado, sliced

- Salsa (optional)

Instructions:

1. Blanch collard green leaves in hot water for 1-2 minutes to soften.

2. In a skillet, cook ground turkey with cumin, paprika, salt, and pepper until browned.

3. Lay out collard green leaves and add a scoop of the turkey mixture.

4. Top with avocado slices and salsa if desired.

5. Roll the collard leaves to form wraps and secure with toothpicks if needed.

5. Lettuce Wrap Tacos with Ground Turkey

A taco feast without the traditional tortillas! Ground turkey seasoned with herbs and spices is nestled into crisp lettuce leaves, creating a light yet flavorful lunch for blood type O individuals.

Ingredients:

- Iceberg lettuce leaves

- 1/2 lb lean ground turkey

- 1 teaspoon chili powder

- 1/2 teaspoon cumin

- Salt and pepper to taste

- Tomatoes, diced

- Red onion, finely chopped

- Fresh cilantro, chopped

- Guacamole (optional)

Instructions:

1. In a skillet, cook ground turkey with chili powder, cumin, salt, and pepper until cooked through.

2. Arrange iceberg lettuce leaves on a plate.

3. Spoon the ground turkey mixture onto each lettuce leaf.

4. Top with diced tomatoes, red onion, and fresh cilantro.

5. Serve with a side of guacamole if desired.

6. Lemon Garlic Shrimp Stir-Fry

A vibrant stir-fry featuring succulent shrimp infused with the flavors of lemon and garlic. Paired with a colorful array of vegetables, this dish provides a delicious and protein-rich lunch option.

Ingredients:

- 1/2 lb shrimp, peeled and deveined

- 2 tablespoons olive oil

- 2 cloves garlic, minced

- Zest of 1 lemon

- 1 teaspoon dried thyme

- Mixed vegetables (bell peppers, broccoli, snap peas)

- Salt and pepper to taste

Instructions:

1. In a wok or skillet, heat olive oil over medium-high heat.

2. Add minced garlic, lemon zest, and dried thyme. Sauté for 1-2 minutes.

3. Add shrimp and cook until pink and opaque.

4. Toss in mixed vegetables and stir-fry until crisp-tender.

5. Season with salt and pepper. Serve hot.

7. Avocado and Chickpea Salad

Creamy avocados and hearty chickpeas come together in a refreshing salad. Tossed with a lemon vinaigrette and fresh herbs, this salad makes for a satisfying and nutrient-dense lunch.

Ingredients:

- 1 can (15 oz) chickpeas, drained and rinsed

- 1 avocado, diced

- Cherry tomatoes, halved

- Cucumber, diced

- Red onion, finely chopped

- Fresh cilantro, chopped

- Olive oil and lemon juice dressing

Instructions:

1. In a large bowl, combine chickpeas, diced avocado, cherry tomatoes, cucumber, red onion, and cilantro.

2. Drizzle with olive oil and lemon juice dressing. Toss gently.

3. Serve as a refreshing and nutritious salad.

8. Quinoa and Spinach Stuffed Peppers

Colorful bell peppers are filled with a wholesome mixture of quinoa and sautéed spinach. Baked to perfection, these stuffed peppers offer a tasty and plant-based lunch option for blood type O individuals.

Ingredients:

- Bell peppers (assorted colors)

- 1 cup cooked quinoa

- Fresh spinach, chopped

- Feta cheese, crumbled

- Cherry tomatoes, diced

- Olive oil

- Salt and pepper to taste

Instructions:

1. Preheat the oven to 375°F (190°C).

2. Cut the tops off the bell peppers and remove seeds.

3. In a bowl, mix cooked quinoa, chopped spinach, feta cheese, diced cherry tomatoes, olive oil, salt, and pepper.

4. Stuff each bell pepper with the quinoa mixture.

5. Bake for 25-30 minutes or until peppers are tender.

9. Lentil and Kale Soup

A hearty soup combining protein-rich lentils with nutrient-packed kale. Seasoned with herbs and spices, this comforting soup is a flavorful and filling lunch choice.

Ingredients:

- 1 cup dry green lentils, rinsed

- 4 cups vegetable broth

- 1 onion, diced

- 2 carrots, sliced

- 2 celery stalks, chopped

- 2 cups kale, chopped

- 2 cloves garlic, minced

- 1 teaspoon cumin

- Salt and pepper to taste

Instructions:

1. In a large pot, combine lentils, vegetable broth, onion, carrots, celery, garlic, cumin, salt, and pepper.

2. Bring to a boil, then reduce heat and simmer for 20-25 minutes.

3. Add chopped kale and simmer for an additional 5 minutes.

4. Adjust seasoning as needed. Serve hot.

10. Baked Lemon Herb Chicken with Sweet Potato

Baked chicken infused with lemon and aromatic herbs, served alongside roasted sweet potato wedges. This meal provides a balance of protein and complex carbohydrates, making it a satisfying and nutritious lunch option.

Ingredients:

- 2 boneless, skinless chicken breasts

- 1 tablespoon olive oil

- Zest of 1 lemon

- 1 teaspoon dried rosemary

- 2 sweet potatoes, sliced

- Salt and pepper to taste

Instructions:

1. Preheat the oven to 400°F (200°C).

2. In a bowl, mix olive oil, lemon zest, dried rosemary, salt, and pepper.

3. Coat chicken breasts with the herb mixture.

4. Place chicken breasts and sweet potato slices on a baking sheet.

5. Bake for 25-30 minutes or until chicken is cooked through and sweet potatoes are tender.

Chapter 3: Dinner Delicacies

1. Rosemary Garlic Roast Beef

A classic roast beef dish infused with the bold flavors of rosemary and garlic. This protein-packed main course is perfect for a special dinner, served alongside roasted vegetables for a wholesome meal.

Ingredients:

- 2 lbs beef roast (such as sirloin or tenderloin)

- 3 cloves garlic, minced

- 2 tablespoons fresh rosemary, chopped

- Salt and pepper to taste

- Olive oil for searing

Instructions:

1. Preheat the oven to 375°F (190°C).

2. Rub the beef roast with minced garlic, chopped rosemary, salt, and pepper.

3. In a skillet, heat olive oil over medium-high heat.

4. Sear the beef on all sides until browned.

5. Transfer the beef to a roasting pan and roast in the oven for about 25-30 minutes for medium-rare or longer if desired.

6. Let it rest before slicing. Serve with roasted vegetables.

2. Lemon Herb Grilled Swordfish

Succulent swordfish steaks marinated in a zesty blend of lemon and herbs, grilled to perfection. This dinner option is rich in omega-3 fatty acids, offering a light and flavorful seafood experience.

Ingredients:

- 2 swordfish steaks

- 1/4 cup olive oil

- Zest and juice of 1 lemon

- 2 cloves garlic, minced

- 1 teaspoon dried oregano

- Salt and pepper to taste

Instructions:

1. In a bowl, whisk together olive oil, lemon zest, lemon juice, minced garlic, dried oregano, salt, and pepper.

2. Place swordfish steaks in a dish and pour the marinade over them. Let marinate for at least 30 minutes.

3. Preheat the grill to medium-high heat.

4. Grill the swordfish for about 4-5 minutes per side or until cooked through.

5. Serve with a side of grilled vegetables.

3. Turkey and Quinoa Stuffed Bell Peppers

Colorful bell peppers stuffed with a delightful mixture of lean ground turkey, quinoa, and a medley of vegetables. Baked until tender, these stuffed peppers provide a satisfying and nutritionally balanced dinner.

Ingredients:

- 4 bell peppers, halved and seeds removed

- 1 lb lean ground turkey

- 1 cup cooked quinoa

- 1 onion, diced

- 2 cloves garlic, minced

- 1 can (14 oz) diced tomatoes

- 1 teaspoon dried oregano

- Salt and pepper to taste

- Shredded cheese for topping (optional)

Instructions:

1. Preheat the oven to 375°F (190°C).

2. In a skillet, cook ground turkey until browned. Add diced onion and garlic, cooking until softened.

3. Stir in cooked quinoa, diced tomatoes, dried oregano, salt, and pepper.

4. Spoon the turkey mixture into halved bell peppers.

5. Top with shredded cheese if desired.

6. Bake for 25-30 minutes or until the peppers are tender.

4. Chicken and Broccoli Stir-Fry

A quick and healthy stir-fry featuring tender chicken pieces, crisp broccoli, and an assortment of colorful vegetables. The savory sauce enhances the flavors, making it a delicious and nutritious dinner choice.

Ingredients:

- 1 lb boneless, skinless chicken breast, thinly sliced

- 2 cups broccoli florets

- 1 bell pepper, thinly sliced

- 2 tablespoons soy sauce

- 1 tablespoon oyster sauce

- 1 teaspoon sesame oil

- 2 cloves garlic, minced

- 1 teaspoon ginger, grated

- 2 tablespoons vegetable oil

Instructions:

1. In a bowl, mix soy sauce, oyster sauce, and sesame oil.

2. Heat vegetable oil in a wok or skillet over high heat.

3. Add sliced chicken and stir-fry until browned and cooked through.

4. Add minced garlic and grated ginger, stir-fry for 1-2 minutes.

5. Add broccoli and bell pepper, continue to stir-fry until vegetables are crisp-tender.

6. Pour the sauce over the stir-fry and toss until everything is well coated.

7. Serve hot over brown rice or quinoa.

5. Baked Salmon with Dill and Asparagus

Salmon fillets baked to perfection with a dill-infused marinade, accompanied by roasted asparagus. This dinner option not only delivers a burst of flavors but also provides a healthy dose of omega-3 fatty acids.

Ingredients:

- 4 salmon fillets

- 1/4 cup olive oil

- Zest and juice of 1 lemon

- 2 tablespoons fresh dill, chopped

- Salt and pepper to taste

- 1 lb asparagus, trimmed

Instructions:

1. Preheat the oven to 375°F (190°C).

2. In a bowl, whisk together olive oil, lemon zest, lemon juice, chopped dill, salt, and pepper.

3. Place salmon fillets on a baking sheet and arrange asparagus around them.

4. Pour the marinade over the salmon and asparagus.

5. Bake for 15-20 minutes or until the salmon flakes easily with a fork.

6. Serve hot, garnished with additional fresh dill.

6. Mediterranean Shrimp Skewers

Juicy shrimp skewers marinated in Mediterranean-inspired flavors, including olive oil, garlic, and herbs. Grilled to perfection, these skewers offer a taste of the Mediterranean for a light and satisfying dinner.

Ingredients:

- 1 lb large shrimp, peeled and deveined

- 1/4 cup olive oil

- 2 cloves garlic, minced

- 1 teaspoon dried oregano

- 1 lemon, sliced

- Cherry tomatoes

- Red onion, cut into chunks

- Wooden skewers, soaked in water

Instructions:

1. In a bowl, mix olive oil, minced garlic, and dried oregano.

2. Thread shrimp, lemon slices, cherry tomatoes, and red onion onto the soaked skewers.

3. Brush the skewers with the olive oil mixture.

4. Grill for 2-3 minutes per side or until the shrimp is opaque.

5. Serve over a bed of quinoa or with a side of Greek salad.

7. Quinoa and Black Bean Bowl

A hearty and nutritious bowl featuring quinoa, black beans, and an array of colorful vegetables. Topped with creamy avocado and a zesty lime dressing, this plant-based dinner is both satisfying and flavorful.

Ingredients:

- 1 cup cooked quinoa

- 1 can (15 oz) black beans, drained and rinsed

- 1 cup cherry tomatoes, halved

- 1 cucumber, diced

- 1 avocado, diced

- Fresh cilantro, chopped

- Olive oil and lime dressing

Instructions:

1. In a bowl, combine cooked quinoa, black beans, cherry tomatoes, cucumber, and avocado.

2. Drizzle with olive oil and lime dressing. Toss gently.

3. Garnish with fresh cilantro. Serve as a nutritious and satisfying bowl.

8. Beef and Vegetable Stir-Fry with Ginger

Thinly sliced beef stir-fried with a vibrant assortment of fresh vegetables and a ginger-infused sauce. This quick and flavorful dinner option is a delightful combination of protein and nutrient-rich vegetables.

Ingredients:

- 1 lb flank steak, thinly sliced

- 2 cups broccoli florets

- 1 red bell pepper, sliced

- 1 yellow bell pepper, sliced

- 3 tablespoons soy sauce

- 1 tablespoon oyster sauce

- 1 tablespoon fresh ginger, grated

- 2 cloves garlic, minced

- 2 tablespoons vegetable oil

Instructions:

1. In a bowl, mix soy sauce, oyster sauce, grated ginger, and minced garlic.

2. Heat vegetable oil in a wok or skillet over high heat.

3. Stir-fry sliced beef until browned, then add broccoli and bell peppers.

4. Continue to stir-fry until vegetables are tender-crisp.

5. Pour the sauce over the stir-fry and toss until well-coated.

6. Serve over brown rice or cauliflower rice.

9. Grilled Lemon Herb Chicken with Sweet Potato Wedges

Chicken marinated in a refreshing blend of lemon and herbs, grilled to perfection, and served alongside baked sweet potato wedges. This dinner dish offers a harmonious mix of flavors and nutrients.

Ingredients:

- 2 boneless, skinless chicken breasts

- 1/4 cup olive oil

- Zest and juice of 1 lemon

- 1 tablespoon fresh thyme, chopped

- 2 sweet potatoes, cut into wedges

- Salt and pepper to taste

Instructions:

1. In a bowl, whisk together olive oil, lemon zest, lemon juice, and chopped thyme.

2. Coat chicken breasts with the marinade and let sit for 30 minutes.

3. Preheat the grill or oven to medium-high heat.

4. Grill or bake chicken until cooked through.

5. Toss sweet potato wedges in olive oil, salt, and pepper, then grill or bake until golden.

6. Serve the chicken over a bed of sweet potato wedges.

10. Lentil and Spinach Curry

A warming and flavorful lentil curry with the addition of nutrient-rich spinach. Infused with aromatic spices, this plant-based dinner is served over brown rice for a satisfying and wholesome meal.

Ingredients:

- 1 cup dry green lentils, rinsed

- 1 onion, finely chopped

- 2 tomatoes, diced

- 2 cups spinach, chopped

- 2 cloves garlic, minced

- 1 tablespoon curry powder

- 1 teaspoon cumin

- 1 teaspoon turmeric

- Salt and pepper to taste

- 2 tablespoons olive oil

Instructions:

1. Cook lentils according to package instructions.

2. In a skillet, heat olive oil and sauté chopped onion until softened.

3. Add minced garlic and diced tomatoes, cook until tomatoes are softened.

4. Stir in curry powder, cumin, turmeric, salt, and pepper.

5. Add cooked lentils and chopped spinach, cook until spinach wilts.

6. Adjust seasoning as needed. Serve over brown rice.

Chapter 4: Snack Attack

1. Nutty Trail Mix

A satisfying blend of blood type O-friendly nuts such as walnuts, almonds, and pistachios, mixed with dried cranberries or cherries. This nutrient-packed trail mix provides a delicious energy boost for on-the-go snacking.

Ingredients:

- 1 cup walnuts

- 1 cup almonds

- 1/2 cup pistachios

- 1/2 cup dried cranberries or cherries

Instructions:

1. In a bowl, combine walnuts, almonds, pistachios, and dried cranberries or cherries.

2. Mix well and portion into snack-sized servings.

3. Enjoy as a quick and energizing trail mix.

2. Greek Yogurt Parfait

Layered Greek yogurt with fresh berries, sliced almonds, and a drizzle of honey. This parfait is not only rich in protein but also offers a mix of textures and flavors for a delightful and wholesome snack.

Ingredients:

- 1 cup Greek yogurt

- 1/2 cup fresh berries (blueberries, strawberries, or raspberries)

- 2 tablespoons sliced almonds

- 1 tablespoon honey

Instructions:

1. In a glass or bowl, layer Greek yogurt with fresh berries.

2. Sprinkle sliced almonds on top.

3. Drizzle honey over the parfait.

4. Repeat layers if desired.

5. Enjoy this protein-packed and flavorful yogurt parfait.

3. Rice Cake with Almond Butter and Banana

A crunchy rice cake spread with almond butter and topped with banana slices. This simple and satisfying snack provides a balance of carbohydrates, healthy fats, and potassium.

Ingredients:

- 1 rice cake

- 2 tablespoons almond butter

- 1/2 banana, sliced

Instructions:

1. Spread almond butter over the rice cake.

2. Arrange banana slices on top.

3. Enjoy this crunchy and satisfying snack.

4. Avocado and Tomato Salsa

Fresh avocado slices paired with a zesty tomato salsa made with diced tomatoes, red onion, cilantro, and a squeeze of lime juice. This snack is both delicious and packed with nutrients.

Ingredients:

- 1 ripe avocado, sliced

- 1 cup diced tomatoes

- 1/4 cup finely chopped red onion

- 2 tablespoons fresh cilantro, chopped

- Juice of 1 lime

- Salt and pepper to taste

Instructions:

1. In a bowl, combine sliced avocado, diced tomatoes, red onion, and cilantro.

2. Squeeze lime juice over the mixture and gently toss.

3. Season with salt and pepper.

4. Enjoy this fresh and nutrient-packed avocado salsa with whole-grain chips or veggie sticks.

5. Cottage Cheese with Pineapple

Creamy cottage cheese served with chunks of fresh pineapple. This snack offers a combination of protein and natural sweetness, making it a refreshing and filling option.

Ingredients:

- 1 cup cottage cheese

- 1 cup fresh pineapple chunks

Instructions:

1. In a bowl, combine cottage cheese with fresh pineapple chunks.

2. Mix gently.

3. Enjoy this creamy and sweet snack that provides a combination of protein and natural sweetness.

6. Hard-Boiled Eggs with Hummus

Hard-boiled eggs paired with a side of hummus for a protein-rich and satisfying snack. The combination of textures and flavors makes this a tasty and nutritious choice.

Ingredients:

- 2 hard-boiled eggs

- 1/4 cup hummus

Instructions:

1. Peel the hard-boiled eggs and slice them in half.

2. Serve with a side of hummus for dipping.

3. Enjoy this protein-rich and satisfying snack.

7. Veggie Sticks with Guacamole

Colorful vegetable sticks, such as carrots, celery, and bell peppers, served with homemade guacamole. This snack provides a mix of crunchy vegetables and the creamy goodness of avocado.

Ingredients:

- Assorted vegetable sticks (carrots, celery, bell peppers)

- 1 ripe avocado

- 1 small tomato, diced

- 1/4 cup red onion, finely chopped

- 1 tablespoon fresh cilantro, chopped

- Juice of 1 lime

- Salt and pepper to taste

Instructions:

1. Cut the vegetables into sticks.

2. In a bowl, mash the ripe avocado and mix in diced tomato, red onion, cilantro, lime juice, salt, and pepper.

3. Serve the veggie sticks with guacamole for a tasty and nutrient-rich snack.

8. Chia Seed Pudding

Chia seeds soaked in almond milk or coconut milk, flavored with a touch of vanilla, and topped with sliced strawberries or blueberries. This pudding is a nutrient-dense and satisfying treat.

Ingredients:

- 1/4 cup chia seeds

- 1 cup almond milk or coconut milk

- 1/2 teaspoon vanilla extract

- Fresh berries for topping

Instructions:

1. In a jar, mix chia seeds, almond milk or coconut milk, and vanilla extract.

2. Stir well and refrigerate for at least 2 hours or overnight until it thickens.

3. Top with fresh berries before serving.

4. Enjoy this chia seed pudding for a nutrient-dense and satisfying snack.

9. Smoked Salmon Roll-Ups

Smoked salmon slices wrapped around cucumber spears and a smear of cream cheese. These roll-ups offer a combination of omega-3 fatty acids, protein, and a refreshing crunch.

Ingredients:

- Smoked salmon slices

- Cucumber spears

- Cream cheese

Instructions:

1. Lay out smoked salmon slices.

2. Spread a thin layer of cream cheese on each slice.

3. Place a cucumber spear at one end and roll up the salmon slice.

4. Secure with a toothpick if needed.

5. Enjoy these elegant and omega-3 rich salmon roll-ups.

10. Almond and Date Energy Bites

Homemade energy bites made with a blend of almonds, dates, and a hint of cinnamon. These bite-sized snacks are perfect for a quick burst of energy without compromising on nutritional value.

Ingredients:

- 1 cup almonds

- 1 cup dates, pitted

- 1/2 teaspoon cinnamon

- Pinch of sea salt

Instructions:

1. In a food processor, blend almonds until finely chopped.

2. Add dates, cinnamon, and a pinch of sea salt. Blend until the mixture sticks together.

3. Roll the mixture into bite-sized balls.

4. Refrigerate for at least 30 minutes before serving.

5. Enjoy these energy bites for a naturally sweet and satisfying snack.

Chapter 5: Sweet Indulgences

1. Dark Chocolate-Covered Almonds

Whole almonds coated in rich, dark chocolate. This treat provides a satisfying combination of healthy fats, antioxidants, and a delightful crunch.

Ingredients:

- 1 cup whole almonds

- 1/2 cup dark chocolate chips or chopped dark chocolate

Instructions:

1. Melt the dark chocolate in a heatproof bowl over simmering water or in the microwave.

2. Dip each almond into the melted chocolate, coating it evenly.

3. Place the chocolate-covered almonds on a parchment paper-lined tray.

4. Allow them to cool and harden.

5. Store in an airtight container.

2. Berry and Nut Smoothie Bowl

A smoothie bowl made with blood type O-friendly berries (such as blueberries and strawberries) and topped with chopped nuts, shredded coconut, and a drizzle of honey. This indulgent bowl is a nutritious and visually appealing dessert.

Ingredients:

- 1 cup mixed berries (blueberries, strawberries)

- 1 banana, frozen

- 1/2 cup Greek yogurt

- 1/4 cup chopped nuts (almonds, walnuts)

- 2 tablespoons shredded coconut

- 1 tablespoon honey

Instructions:

1. In a blender, combine the mixed berries, frozen banana, and Greek yogurt. Blend until smooth.

2. Pour the smoothie into a bowl.

3. Top with chopped nuts, shredded coconut, and a drizzle of honey.

4. Enjoy this visually appealing and nutritious dessert.

3. Banana Almond Butter Bites

Sliced bananas topped with a dollop of almond butter and a sprinkle of cinnamon. These bite-sized treats offer a perfect blend of sweetness and healthy fats.

Ingredients:

- 2 bananas, sliced

- 1/4 cup almond butter

- Cinnamon for sprinkling

Instructions:

1. Lay banana slices on a plate or tray.

2. Place a small dollop of almond butter on each banana slice.

3. Sprinkle with cinnamon.

4. Enjoy these bite-sized banana almond butter bites.

4. Coconut Chia Pudding

A creamy chia seed pudding made with coconut milk, sweetened with a touch of honey or maple syrup, and topped with fresh tropical fruits. This dessert is rich in omega-3 fatty acids and provides a satisfying texture.

Ingredients:

- 1/4 cup chia seeds

- 1 cup coconut milk

- 1 tablespoon honey or maple syrup

- Fresh tropical fruits for topping (mango, pineapple)

Instructions:

1. In a bowl, mix chia seeds, coconut milk, and honey or maple syrup.

2. Stir well and refrigerate for at least 2 hours or overnight until it thickens.

3. Top with fresh tropical fruits before serving.

4. Enjoy this creamy and omega-3 rich coconut chia pudding.

5. Greek Yogurt with Honey and Walnuts

Thick Greek yogurt drizzled with raw honey and topped with chopped walnuts. This simple yet decadent dessert offers a balance of creamy, sweet, and crunchy elements.

Ingredients:

- 1 cup Greek yogurt

- 2 tablespoons raw honey

- 1/4 cup chopped walnuts

Instructions:

1. Spoon Greek yogurt into a serving dish.

2. Drizzle with raw honey.

3. Sprinkle chopped walnuts on top.

4. Enjoy this simple and decadent Greek yogurt dessert.

6. Baked Apples with Cinnamon

Sliced apples baked with a sprinkle of cinnamon until tender. This warm and comforting dessert is a healthier alternative to traditional apple pie.

Ingredients:

- 4 apples, cored and sliced

- 1 teaspoon cinnamon

- 1 tablespoon honey

Instructions:

1. Preheat the oven to 375°F (190°C).

2. In a bowl, toss apple slices with cinnamon and honey.

3. Spread the apples in a baking dish.

4. Bake for 20-25 minutes or until tender.

5. Serve warm for a comforting and naturally sweet dessert.

7. Frozen Banana Pops

Banana slices dipped in dark chocolate and frozen until solid. These frozen banana pops make for a refreshing and naturally sweet treat.

Ingredients:

- 2 bananas, peeled and cut in half

- 1/2 cup dark chocolate chips

- 2 tablespoons chopped nuts (pistachios, almonds)

Instructions:

1. Insert a popsicle stick into each banana half.

2. Melt the dark chocolate in a heatproof bowl.

3. Dip each banana into the melted chocolate and sprinkle with chopped nuts.

4. Place on a parchment paper-lined tray and freeze until solid.

5. Enjoy these refreshing and chocolaty frozen banana pops.

8. Pomegranate and Pistachio Parfait

Layers of fresh pomegranate seeds, Greek yogurt, and chopped pistachios. This parfait is not only visually appealing but also provides a burst of antioxidants and healthy fats.

Ingredients:

- 1 cup pomegranate seeds

- 1 cup Greek yogurt

- 2 tablespoons chopped pistachios

- 1 tablespoon honey

Instructions:

1. In a glass or bowl, layer pomegranate seeds with Greek yogurt.

2. Sprinkle chopped pistachios on top.

3. Drizzle with honey.

4. Repeat layers if desired.

5. Enjoy this antioxidant-rich and indulgent parfait.

9. Almond Flour Blueberry Muffins

Moist and fluffy blueberry muffins made with almond flour, sweetened with a touch of honey or agave nectar. These muffins are gluten-free and suitable for blood type O individuals.

Ingredients:

- 2 cups almond flour

- 1/2 teaspoon baking soda

- 1/4 teaspoon salt

- 3 eggs

- 1/4 cup honey or agave nectar

- 1/4 cup coconut oil, melted

- 1 teaspoon vanilla extract

- 1 cup blueberries

Instructions:

1. Preheat the oven to 350°F (175°C). Line a muffin tin with paper liners.

2. In a bowl, mix almond flour, baking soda, and salt.

3. In another bowl, whisk together eggs, honey, melted coconut oil, and vanilla extract.

4. Combine wet and dry ingredients, then fold in blueberries.

5. Divide the batter into muffin cups and bake for 20-25 minutes.

6. Enjoy these moist and naturally sweet almond flour blueberry muffins.

10. Chocolate Avocado Mousse

A velvety chocolate mousse made with ripe avocados, cocoa powder, and a sweetener like maple syrup. This indulgent dessert is rich in healthy fats and satisfies chocolate cravings.

Ingredients:

- 2 ripe avocados

- 1/4 cup cocoa powder

- 1/4 cup maple syrup

- 1 teaspoon vanilla extract

- Pinch of salt

- Fresh berries for garnish

Instructions:

1. In a blender, combine avocados, cocoa powder, maple syrup, vanilla extract, and a pinch of salt.

2. Blend until smooth and creamy.

3. Chill the mousse in the refrigerator for at least 30 minutes.

4. Serve topped with fresh berries for a decadent chocolate avocado mousse.

Chapter 6: Beverages and Smoothies

1. Berry Blast Smoothie

A vibrant blend of blood type O-friendly berries such as blueberries, strawberries, and raspberries. Mix with almond milk, a scoop of protein powder, and a touch of honey for a refreshing and protein-packed smoothie.

Ingredients:

- 1 cup blueberries

- 1/2 cup strawberries, hulled

- 1/2 cup raspberries

- 1 scoop protein powder

- 1 cup almond milk

- 1 tablespoon honey

Instructions:

1. In a blender, combine blueberries, strawberries, raspberries, protein powder, and almond milk.

2. Blend until smooth.

3. Add honey for sweetness and blend again.

4. Pour into a glass and enjoy this protein-packed Berry Blast Smoothie.

2. Green Machine Smoothie

A nutrient-packed smoothie featuring kale or spinach, cucumber, green apple, and a tablespoon of chia seeds. Blend with water or coconut water for a hydrating and detoxifying green smoothie.

Ingredients:

- 1 cup kale or spinach, stems removed

- 1/2 cucumber, peeled and sliced

- 1 green apple, cored and sliced

- 1 tablespoon chia seeds

- 1 cup water or coconut water

Instructions:

1. Place kale or spinach, cucumber, green apple, and chia seeds in a blender.

2. Add water or coconut water.

3. Blend until smooth.

4. Pour into a glass and enjoy the nutrient-packed Green Machine Smoothie.

3. Pineapple Mint Cooler

A tropical refreshment combining pineapple chunks, fresh mint leaves, and coconut water. This cooling beverage is perfect for a hot day and provides a naturally sweet taste without citrus.

Ingredients:

- 1 cup pineapple chunks

- Handful of fresh mint leaves

- 1 cup coconut water

- Ice cubes

Instructions:

1. In a blender, combine pineapple chunks, fresh mint leaves, and coconut water.

2. Blend until smooth.

3. Add ice cubes and blend again until well combined.

4. Pour into a glass and enjoy this tropical Pineapple Mint Cooler.

4. Banana-Berry Protein Shake

A satisfying protein shake made with ripe bananas, mixed berries, almond milk, and a scoop of protein powder. This smoothie offers a creamy texture and a balance of carbohydrates and protein.

Ingredients:

- 2 ripe bananas

- 1/2 cup mixed berries (blueberries, strawberries)

- 1 cup almond milk

- 1 scoop protein powder

Instructions:

1. In a blender, combine ripe bananas, mixed berries, almond milk, and protein powder.

2. Blend until smooth.

3. Pour into a glass and savor the creamy and protein-packed Banana-Berry Protein Shake.

5. Chocolate Almond Joy Smoothie

Indulge in a chocolate treat with this smoothie made from almond milk, cocoa powder, almond butter, and a sprinkle of shredded coconut. A guilt-free pleasure for chocolate lovers.

Ingredients:

- 1 cup almond milk

- 2 tablespoons cocoa powder

- 2 tablespoons almond butter

- 1 tablespoon shredded coconut

- Ice cubes

Instructions:

1. In a blender, combine almond milk, cocoa powder, almond butter, and shredded coconut.

2. Add ice cubes and blend until smooth.

3. Pour into a glass and enjoy this indulgent Chocolate Almond Joy Smoothie.

6. Watermelon Basil Refresher

A hydrating and flavorful drink made with fresh watermelon cubes and a hint of basil. Blend with ice for a refreshing beverage that is perfect for warm days.

Ingredients:

- 2 cups fresh watermelon cubes

- Handful of fresh basil leaves

- Ice cubes

Instructions:

1. In a blender, combine fresh watermelon cubes and basil leaves.

2. Blend until smooth.

3. Add ice cubes and blend again until well combined.

4. Pour into a glass and enjoy this hydrating Watermelon Basil Refresher.

7. Avocado Spinach Smoothie

A creamy green smoothie featuring avocado, spinach, banana, and almond milk. This smoothie is rich in healthy fats and provides a nutrient boost to your day.

Ingredients:

- 1 ripe avocado

- 1 cup spinach leaves

- 1 banana

- 1 cup almond milk

Instructions:

1. In a blender, combine ripe avocado, spinach leaves, banana, and almond milk.

2. Blend until smooth.

3. Pour into a glass and savor the creamy and nutrient-rich Avocado Spinach Smoothie.

8. Cherry Almond Smoothie

Blend together sweet cherries, almond milk, a handful of almonds, and a touch of vanilla extract for a delicious and antioxidant-rich smoothie.

Ingredients:

- 1 cup sweet cherries, pitted

- 1/2 cup almonds

- 1 cup almond milk

- 1/2 teaspoon vanilla extract

Instructions:

1. In a blender, combine sweet cherries, almonds, almond milk, and vanilla extract.

2. Blend until smooth.

3. Pour into a glass and enjoy the delicious and antioxidant-rich Cherry Almond Smoothie.

9. Beetroot Berry Elixir

A vibrant elixir combining beetroot, mixed berries, and coconut water. This antioxidant-packed drink not only looks beautiful but also promotes overall well-being.

Ingredients:

- 1 small beetroot, peeled and chopped

- 1 cup mixed berries (blueberries, raspberries)

- 1 cup coconut water

Instructions:

1. In a blender, combine chopped beetroot, mixed berries, and coconut water.

2. Blend until smooth.

3. Pour into a glass and enjoy this vibrant and antioxidant-packed Beetroot Berry Elixir.

10. Cucumber Mint Cooler

A refreshing cooler made with cucumber slices, fresh mint leaves, and coconut water. This hydrating beverage is perfect for cleansing and rejuvenating your system.

Ingredients:

- 1 cucumber, peeled and sliced

- Handful of fresh mint leaves

- 1 cup coconut water

- Ice cubes

Instructions:

1. In a blender, combine cucumber slices, fresh mint leaves, and coconut water.

2. Blend until smooth.

3. Add ice cubes and blend again until well combined.

4. Pour into a glass and enjoy this refreshing Cucumber Mint Cooler.

14-Day Meal Plan

Day 1

Breakfast: Omelette Extravaganza

Lunch: Grilled Lemon Herb Chicken Bowl

Dinner: Rosemary Garlic Roast Beef

Day 2

Breakfast: Energizing Smoothie Bowl

Lunch: Teriyaki Salmon Quinoa Bowl

Dinner: Lemon Herb Grilled Swordfish

Day 3

Breakfast: Quinoa and Spinach Muffins

Lunch: Greek Salad with Grilled Chicken

Dinner: Turkey and Quinoa Stuffed Bell Peppers

- Stuffed bell peppers with ground turkey, quinoa, and vegetables

Day 4

Breakfast: Tropical Green Power Bowl

Lunch: Turkey and Avocado Collard Wraps

Dinner: Chicken and Broccoli Stir-Fry

Day 5

Breakfast: Almond Flour Banana Muffins

Lunch: Lettuce Wrap Tacos with Ground Turkey

Dinner: Baked Salmon with Dill and Asparagus

Day 6

Breakfast: Berry Blast Breakfast Bowl

Lunch: Lemon Garlic Shrimp Stir-Fry

Dinner: Mediterranean Shrimp Skewers

Day 7

Breakfast: Lemon Garlic Chicken Bowl

Lunch: Avocado and Chickpea Salad

Dinner: Quinoa and Black Bean Bowl

Day 8

Breakfast: Spinach and Feta Breakfast Wrap

Lunch: Quinoa and Spinach Stuffed Peppers

Dinner: Beef and Vegetable Stir-Fry with Ginger

Day 9

Breakfast: Lemon Garlic Chicken Bowl

Lunch: Lentil and Kale Soup

Dinner: Grilled Lemon Herb Chicken with Sweet Potato
Wedges

Day 10

Breakfast: Teriyaki Salmon Quinoa Bowl

Lunch: Baked Lemon Herb Chicken with Sweet Potato

Dinner: Lemon Herb Grilled Swordfish

Day 11

Breakfast: Quinoa and Spinach Muffins

Lunch: Quinoa and Black Bean Bowl

Dinner: Rosemary Garlic Roast Beef

Day 12

Breakfast: Berry Blast Breakfast Bowl

Lunch: Avocado and Chickpea Salad

Dinner: Mediterranean Shrimp Skewers

Day 13

Breakfast: Almond Flour Banana Muffins

Lunch: Lettuce Wrap Tacos with Ground Turkey

Dinner: Beef and Vegetable Stir-Fry with Ginger

Day 14

Breakfast: Lemon Garlic Chicken Bowl

Lunch: Lentil and Kale Soup

Dinner: Grilled Lemon Herb Chicken with Sweet Potato Wedges

Conclusion

The Blood Type O Diet Cookbook serves as a comprehensive guide to crafting a culinary journey that aligns with the nutritional needs of individuals with blood type O. Beyond being a mere collection of recipes, it stands as a testament to the belief that food is not only nourishment for the body but a source of joy, vitality, and well-being.

Through a meticulous curation of diverse recipes, this cookbook endeavors to transform each meal into a delightful experience while adhering to the principles of the blood type diet. The 14-day meal plan, spanning breakfasts, lunches, and dinners, embraces the richness of whole foods, lean proteins, and vibrant vegetables, reflecting a commitment to a balanced and wholesome diet.

The recipes provided here not only tantalize the taste buds but also cater to the specific dietary considerations of blood type O individuals. From the protein-packed Omelette Extravaganza to the nutrient-rich Teriyaki Salmon Quinoa Bowl and the savory Rosemary Garlic Roast Beef, each dish is a carefully crafted fusion of flavors designed to support optimal health.

However, it is crucial to acknowledge the uniqueness of individual needs and preferences. As such, it is recommended that individuals consult healthcare professionals or registered dietitians before embarking on significant dietary changes. The cookbook is intended as a foundation, inviting readers to personalize their culinary experience, ensuring that it resonates with their tastes, lifestyle, and health goals.

In essence, the Blood Type O Diet Cookbook strives to be more than a compilation of recipes; it aspires to be a companion on the journey toward a healthier, more vibrant life. It encourages a mindful and intentional approach to eating, fostering a deeper connection between individuals and the nourishment they provide to their bodies. May this culinary exploration be both satisfying to the palate and nourishing to the soul, as it contributes to the holistic well-being of those who embrace its principles.

About the author

 Becky Shelby is a passionate advocate for holistic well-being, blending her love for nutrition, health, and lifestyle. With a keen interest in exploring the intersection of dietary choices and individual health, Becky has dedicated herself to researching and understanding how nutrition impacts our bodies, specifically in the context of blood types.

Her journey into the world of nutrition began with a personal quest for optimal health and vitality. Drawing inspiration from her own experiences, Becky has delved into the intricacies of the Blood Type Diet, exploring how tailored nutrition can contribute to overall well-being.

As an author, Becky aims to share her knowledge and insights with a wider audience, simplifying complex nutritional concepts and providing practical guidance for individuals seeking to make informed choices aligned with their blood type. Through her writing, she aspires to empower readers to embark on their own journeys toward a healthier and more balanced lifestyle.

Becky's approach is characterized by a commitment to evidence-based information, an appreciation for diverse dietary needs, and a genuine passion for helping others discover the profound impact of mindful nutrition.

Whether you are new to the concept of blood type-based nutrition or seeking to deepen your understanding, Becky Shelby's work invites you to explore the fascinating and personalized world of the Blood Type Diet.

In addition to her writing, Becky enjoys connecting with her readers through various platforms, sharing tips, recipes, and insights to inspire positive changes in their health and well-being. Her mission is to foster a community of individuals who embrace the transformative power of personalized nutrition on their journey to vibrant health.

My Little Request

If you have gotten to this point, chances are high you have finished this book.

Thank You for Reading My Book!

I love hearing what you have to say.

I need your input to make the next version of this

book and my future books better.

Please take two minutes now to leave a helpful review on Amazon letting me know what you thought of the book

Thanks so much!

- Becky Shelby